Beating The Odds!

Beating The

Odds!

A Guide To

Gaining And Maintaining A

Healthier Eating Lifestyle

For Life

Duanita Norman

Acknowledgements

*Special thanks to my mom, Myra Stafford;
and to my son, Eric Norman for their time
and assistance.*

*Thank you to the men and women whose
healthier eating lifestyles, which I have had
the privilege of being a part of, fostered the
writing of this book.*

Table of Contents

Introduction

A dilemma that we face in our culture is how to gain and maintain a healthier eating lifestyle. There are a multitude of books, blogs, articles and health reports telling us what we should do to create this lifestyle for ourselves. Along with this, there are the many different meal plans, meal delivery services, prepared meals in the grocery store and cold/hot food bars making it easier for us to have access to healthier foods. With all of these resources, it would seem like a healthier eating lifestyle would be fairly easy to achieve.

Well, there are reasons why it is easier said than done. First of all, life is busy and we tend to think about everything else first and our food last. Second, the circumstances and events in our lives play a large role in determining what we eat and drink. In fact, they not only trigger what we put in our bodies; but also, where, when and why we do. Many of us have been down the road of trying to achieve a healthier eating lifestyle, only to return back to our previous eating patterns. Most of the time, this occurs because we don't know how to navigate our eating in the midst of what is going on in our lives.

The purpose of this book is to help you to get off of this roller coaster and plant your feet on solid ground. The principles and insights in these pages will help you to gain and maintain a healthier eating lifestyle, during the circumstances and events that happen in your life. The best part is it will be an eating lifestyle that will work for you.

"Knowledge is Power"

– Francis Bacon

Daily Life

What Are You Eating?

The best place to begin, when it comes to implementing a healthier eating lifestyle, is your home. Start by taking an inventory of what you have in your house:

- What foods are in your refrigerator?

- What foods are in your pantry?

- What foods are in your snack bin?

- What beverages are in your house?

Your home is the place where you can have the most influence over what you eat and drink. A primary way to do this is to be aware of the ingredients in the items that you pick up from the grocery store. There are many times we think the foods we are choosing are healthy, but this may not be the case.

Here are a few ways that you can begin to make healthier choices about the foods you bring into your home:

1) Go natural as much as possible. Make sure the majority of the foods in your meals are meats, vegetables, dairy, whole grains and fruit.

2) Read the labels and ask yourself these questions:

- How much fat, sodium and sugar does the item contain?

- How much of the item contains artificial ingredients?

TIP: Ingredients are listed from the most content to the least content.

3) If the label consists of a lot of ingredients that you cannot pronounce, leave it on the shelf!

4) Minimize the processed foods. Artificial ingredients and the sodium content tend to be high in them.

5) Do most of your shopping around the perimeter of the store (where the healthier foods are housed).

Snack Attack

We have all experienced "snack attacks". This happens when you are eating one of your favorite foods and you just can't get enough of it. It is generally something that gives you comfort and a feeling of contentment. Don't assume this doesn't pertain to you if you snack on healthy foods. Even healthy snacks aren't healthy, if you have too much of them. As the saying goes, "too much of a good thing is not a good thing". Over time, our bodies will pay the price for these overindulgences. So, the question becomes:

"How can you enjoy the snacks you love without overdoing it?"

1) Portion-sized bags. This will help to limit the amount that you eat. Also, with a smaller bag, you may give more thought to what you are doing; since you would have to grab another bag to continue your snacking. When you eat out of a larger bag,

it is much easier to continuously eat your favorite snack.

2) Purchase the "reduced" version of the snack. However, here is a word of caution. Take a look at the nutrients in both items. Just because the item says it is "low fat" and/or "sugar free", does not mean it is healthier than the original one. If the reduced item increases the amount of sugar and/or sodium, it may be beneficial to stick with the original version. Remember to pay attention to the suggested serving size on the package (portion control).

3) Figure out what it is about the snack that causes you to like it so much; then, try to find a healthier replacement. It could be that it is crunchy, or sweet, or crunchy and salty, or sweet and salty. An example of a healthy replacement would be having a sweet and crunchy protein bar, that is low in sugar, instead of caramel covered popcorn.

4) If there is a snack food that you love and it is dangerous for you to have it around your house (lack of self control), then keep it out. For example, if potato chips are a "snack attack" item for you, then don't bring them in your house. Instead, have them as a side item when you buy a sandwich at the deli. This will help with portion control by

limiting the accessibility you have to the snack and lessening the temptation.

The Specialty Drink Craze

Specialty coffees and teas have become very popular and start off the day for a lot of people. Drinks such as café mocha, caramel macchiato, chai tea latte and many more have become the norm. However, along with the wonderful taste of these beverages come quite a few calories due to added sugars, like flavored syrups and whipped cream. There are also the specialty teas and coffees that include alcohol along with these added sugars, such as an Irish coffee. Whatever your drink of choice may be, there are a few things you can do to make it healthier for you:

1) Reduce the number of times you enjoy your drink in a day and within the week.

2) If purchasing the drink from a coffee house that has a website, look at how many calories are in it. On some websites, you can change the drink to fit your calorie,

sugar and /or fat requirements. This enables you to order the drink to your specifications. For example, if your drink has 4 pumps of flavored syrup, try reducing it to 2 pumps of the syrup.

3) If the drink is offered in various sizes, lean towards the smaller quantities; and, stay away from the larger ones.

4) Order the "skinny" version of your drink. This version will tend to have fewer calories, less sugar and/or less fat.

5) If you are adventurous, look online for a healthy recipe and make your favorite drink at home.

The Weather Blues

The weather can have quite an effect on us. How do rainy days and cloudy days affect you? They may have a tendency to make you feel like you are dragging, tired and not motivated to do anything. This is a likely time for you to go for those foods and drinks that give you a temporary mental lift, but from a nutritional standpoint, they don't do much for you. The key is to lean towards foods and drinks that satisfy the mental craving, but also support your healthier eating goals.

1) If it is a specialty coffee or tea, choose the small or medium size and try the lighter version.

2) For the foods that you choose, look at what draws you to them. For example, is it the texture (chewy, crunchy or dense), the taste (salty, sweet, or spicy) or possibly a combination of the two? Once you realize what it is, look for a healthier substitute. Some suggestions are:

- Sweet and salty? Try a protein bar with a combination of nuts and chocolate (preferably dark chocolate).

- Salty and crunchy? Try lightly salted nuts (almonds, walnuts, or peanuts), oat bran pretzels or lightly salted popcorn.

- Sweet and cakey? Try a slice of angel food cake with strawberries on top.

- Sweet and dense? Try having a few pieces of dark chocolate (60% cacao or higher).

REMINDER: Be mindful of the serving size.

Lighten Up

As winter leaves, so do many of the heavier foods that are associated with it. With the advent of the spring season, our foods tend to get lighter. Instead of casseroles and stews, we begin to eat more salads, fruits and lighter meals. In fact some of our favorite fruits are in season such as peaches, watermelons and strawberries.

When foods are lighter, you can forget that they have as many calories as some of the heavier foods that you were eating during the winter season. Be mindful of the following, in order to stay on track:

1) Salads are a warm weather favorite! Be aware of what is put in them and on them. Dried fruit has a high content of sugar, nuts are high in fat and salad dressings can be high in fat, sugar or both. Be conscious of the quantity of these items in your salad. You can minimize the amount of salad dressing used by putting the dressing on the side (not on the salad). Dip the fork into the

dressing and then into the salad. This way you will get a taste of the dressing in each bite.

2) Fruit salads are very refreshing at this time of year, but they can contain a high amount of sugar. For this reason, they should be side items or small desserts; and, not a meal. Even though fruit is healthy, too many sugars are not healthy (even if they are natural ones).

3) It is grilling season! Rubs, spices and marinades taste great on all of our grilled foods. However, try to use low sodium rubs and spices; as well as, marinades that are low in sodium and sugar.

4) Last, but not least, are the warm weather drinks; such as fruit juices, lemonades and iced teas. It is all about watching the calories and sugars (natural and artificial).

Seasonal Cravings

When the seasons are changing from summer to fall, and the weather is getting colder, you may find yourself gravitating towards your comfort foods and drinks. Unfortunately, the tendency is to overindulge in these items through the colder months. Then, when the warmer weather is around the corner, we find ourselves scrambling to lose unwanted pounds. It seems like a vicious cycle, but it doesn't have to be! Combating these cravings is to know why you have them and then deciding what can be done to manage them. During this time, here are some questions to ask yourself:

1) What food/drink is creeping into your diet more often than it should be?

2) What is bringing on the craving (stress, discomfort, habit etc…)?

3) Why this particular food/drink? What about it satisfies your craving (salty, crunchy and/or sweet)?

4) When you have indulged in this pattern before what are the long term effects? How do you feel about these effects?

5) Is there a healthier food/drink that can be substituted for the one you are craving? Is there a lighter version of the food available?

Taking the time to answer these questions will help you get a better understanding of your seasonal cravings. It also helps you to move forward with making healthier choices in your eating lifestyle.

A Daily Equation

Here is an equation to help keep you on track, daily, to becoming a healthier you!

1) Eat well! Limit the amount of processed foods, sugars, fat and sodium.

+

2) Portion Control!

+

3) Water! Hydration is a key element.

+

4) Watch your alcoholic intake!

+

5) Get enough sleep!

_____

A Healthier You!

Busy Life

"To Go, Please"

There are times when you may feel like your life is all over the place! When life goes off course, eating habits can have a tendency to do the same thing. Finding the time to sit down and eat can be difficult. You are "on the go"! So, how do you steady the course when there is limited time to eat and less time to prepare meals? Here are some options for those hectic times:

Breakfast (on the go)

1) Boiled eggs and a slice of dry whole grain/whole wheat toast

2) Fruit (apples, berries or a banana) and nuts (almonds, walnuts, or peanuts)

3) Smoothie or Protein drink

4) Protein bar/ Meal bar

Lunch (on the go)

1) Make a sandwich and add some raw vegetables on the side to take with you.

2) Homemade lunch pack made up of finger foods.

You can create this by taking a sectioned container and packing it with proteins, fruits, vegetables and/or healthy carbs. An example would be slices of cheese, whole wheat crackers, nuts, berries and/or mini bell peppers.

3) Smoothie or protein drink

4) Protein bar/ Meal bar

Dinner

Crock pot/Slow cooker meals

Place your ingredients in the crock pot/slow cooker and turn it to the designated temperature and time (according to your recipe). When it is done, you are ready to eat! You can also place the meal in a container and refrigerate/freeze it. Now you have a quick meal for tomorrow or for a later date.

All In One

Life is busy! There is work, the commute back and forth, your children's after school activities, homework duties in the evening, as well as, the work you brought home from the office. With all of this going on, you have no time to think about what to have for dinner. Unfortunately, when life gets busy, we find ourselves eating dinner out more and grabbing breakfast and lunch "on the go" at fast food restaurants. One solution to staying on track when life gets a little crazy is the "one pot meal".

One pot meals are very convenient! Instead of trying to cook 2 or 3 different foods separately to have a meal, you take a few foods and include them all in one pot. These meals can be prepared in a slow cooker, on the stove or in the oven. Some of them have a lot of ingredients and some have a few ingredients. If you are not familiar with preparing this type of meal, here are some guidelines you can follow:

1) Decide what mode of cooking suits you best (slow cooker, stove, oven).

2) Go online and use the following search terms: "slow cooker meals", "one pot meals on the stove" or "one pot meals in the oven"

3) As you find recipes that you like, begin to make a file for yourself. This will enable you to have the recipes readily available the next time life becomes overwhelming.

Also, these meals are not just for dinner. There are recipes for breakfast, lunch, snacks and desserts. The "one pot meal" is very convenient when you don't have a lot of time. They provide a way for you to stay on track with your healthier eating lifestyle.

Help!

Being disciplined in your eating habits can be a daunting task. With so many things to take care of, you may find yourself needing help. This is where the commercial diet can be of assistance. These are the programs that have been created to help you gain structure in your eating lifestyle, which in turn, can lead you to reaching your healthier eating goals. Some of these programs require the use of their brand of food and drink; whereas, other programs will have you use the brand of your choice. In some cases, it is a combination of what they provide and what you provide. Either way, there are so many options available, that there is one to suit everyone. If this is the path you choose to take, consider the following:

1) A question to ask is, "How long do I plan to participate in this program?" The goal may be to use the program the rest of your life or you may have a specific time frame. It may be until you reach your goal weight

and/or until you have stabilized your eating habits. Having your goal in mind will help you to stay focused and on track.

2) If your plan is to end the program at a certain point, take note of the tools you are using that work for you. When you discontinue the program, you may no longer have access to them. So, begin to devise ways of how you can put these tools into practice on your own. A way that you can go about doing this is to look online for tools that mirror the ones that you are using. This will enable you to stay the course once you have exited the program.

3) If you are on a plan where you are using the food and drink that is provided, look at the nutritional facts and ingredients in them and find similar items in the grocery store. This gives you the option of using your food and/or the food provided by your program.

Snack Box Option

Bento boxes are compartmentalized boxes that are used for carrying meals and snacks. They are convenient and available in many different sizes. Some of these boxes are also equipped with ice packs and bottles for carrying perishable foods and liquids. A few ways that the bento box can be beneficial to your busy life are:

1) If you get stuck in traffic and find yourself getting hungry, you will have nutritious snacks at your fingertips. Fill a box with non-perishable snacks and keep it in the glove compartment of your car. For example, some snacks that could be packed are trail mix, nuts, seeds (sunflower, pumpkin etc...) and a protein bar.

2) You may have a job that involves running from one appointment to another, like an outside sales position. Since the bento box is portable, it is very easy to take your food wherever you go. This can also help you to

27

avoid a trip to the nearest fast food restaurant.

3) These boxes are also great if you travel for work. If you have an unexpected delay and/or you are not able to stop and eat, you will have food on hand. Fill the box with healthy snack foods and put it in your carry-on luggage, lap top bag or briefcase.

As previously mentioned, there are also bento boxes that are made for carrying a meal. Therefore, if you have a lengthy flight, a meal box may be the better option.

A Quick Fix

When life is busy, there are times when you need to grab something that is quick. This is when protein bars and protein drinks can be beneficial. They are quick and easy to carry along with you. In some cases, due to their high nutritional value, they are able to stand in as a substitute for a meal. This is when you may see the term "meal replacement" on the package.

Even though these drinks and bars tend to be healthy, some of them can be high in sugar and artificial sweeteners. When you go to purchase these items, be sure to read the labels. They will provide you with information on all of the nutrients, in order to make an informed decision.

Protein bars can also be an alternative for having a candy bar, if you have a sweet tooth. There are so many varieties that there is bound to be one that will satisfy your craving. This option provides better nutrition and the added benefit of reduced calories.

The Frequent Flyer

Do you travel frequently for work? If so, you are among the many people who do. Most people who travel for work find it very difficult to maintain a healthier eating plan; because, they are in a position where they have limited control over their food choices. In fact, when on travel, eating out becomes the norm. Travelling for work can wreak havoc on a healthier eating lifestyle. However, there are some things that can be done while on travel to maintain your eating habits.

Healthy Eating Tips for the Frequent Flyer

1) When booking a motel/hotel room, try to book one that has a kitchenette. If that is not available, then try to book a room that has a refrigerator. This gives you the ability to have your own snacks and food to eat, instead of relying on what is around you.

2) Book your flight so you arrive a little early. This will give you time to settle in and

visit the local food store to purchase food and drink for some of your meals and/or snacks, to have in your room.

3) Be sure to have healthy snacks on hand when you are attending conferences and meetings. This enables you to have a nutritious snack instead of the cookies, pastries and other snacks that may be available.

4) When eating out, you may be able to choose a healthy option. A lot of places have healthy options available; and, will have a section where they are housed on the menu.

5) When drinking alcohol, be aware of how much you are drinking and; keep in mind, it slows down your metabolism. A good practice is to have a glass of water between drinks. This helps you to reduce your alcohol intake and stay hydrated.

Meals on Wheels

There are many different meals on wheels, aka "home delivery" meal services. This is a concept that has been readily accepted and is welcomed by many. These meals take the thinking out of cooking. The service provides the recipe and a majority of the ingredients, which are delivered to your door for a fee. The only things left for you to do are to open the box, prepare the food and enjoy. Your meals are just a click away on the computer. However, as beneficial as they are, there are a few things to be aware of:

1) These meals can be high in calories. Since they tend to be the dinner meal, it means quite a few calories are being consumed at the end of the day. This is a time when your activity level can begin to wind down. As this happens, your metabolism begins to slow down also. For this reason, when the meal is high in calories, eat half of the meal and save the rest for another day.

2) Watch the sugar content! This ingredient can be high in some of these meals because of how they are prepared. One of the primary ways in which this occurs is when the food includes a sauce or a glaze. Even if it seems like very little is used, pay attention to the nutrition facts to see how much sugar is in each serving.

3) Keep an eye on the sodium levels! Since these foods are packaged and shipped, the sodium content may be high depending on what ingredients are used to preserve them.

TIP: Just as you read the nutrition labels in the grocery store before purchasing, the same thing should be done before making your purchase online.

Stabilizing Life

Stop The Madness!

You spend much of your life managing so many things! You manage your household, your finances, your family, your job, vacations and the list goes on and on. While you take the time to manage all of these areas in life, the one area that tends to get neglected is your eating lifestyle.

A major reason for weight gain is a lack of consciousness about what is going on in your life. Some of the circumstances that can affect you are job changes, children's after school and weekend activities, illness in the family, special occasions, holiday celebrations and stress. When life gets hectic, eating habits tend to adjust to the changes. Unfortunately, these changes can have an adverse effect on your daily diet and also have damaging long term effects.

The key to begin managing weight gain is to recognize when your life is going through changes and be aware of how they can affect your eating. Once you are aware, you can then consider options that are available to help manage this time in your life. Some examples are, making meals in advance, creating meals to take "on the go" and packing healthy snacks.

Management of your eating lifestyle is just as important as all of the other areas of life that you manage.

NOTE: If you seek assistance in this area, reference the previous sections, of this book, entitled "Daily Life and "Busy Life".

Tracking

Tracking calories can be a controversial topic. However, at the end of the day, tracking has proven to be effective in making us more aware of what we are eating and drinking. How long you track your calories is up to you. It can be done for a short period of time or, there are those who will do it for a lifetime. It is contingent on your plan of action for reaching your goals. However long you may decide to be engaged in tracking, here are some benefits to using this tool:

1) With various online systems, when you are tracking your calories, you are also tracking your nutrients. This information is very helpful for maintaining the proper nutrient levels in your diet.

2) How long you track your calories is up to you. If you decide to suspend the tracking, hold on to your information. It may be useful to you in the future. This will be talked about more in point #4.

3) Find a tracking method that works for you. There are many options. It can be written, digital, audible or a combination. A lot of the digital trackers have a function that allows you to scan the bar code of a food in order to record it. With the audible ones, you just speak and it records what you say. These are great options, if you don't want to record your food and drink manually.

4) Your tracking can prove to be very helpful to you in the future, as mentioned in point #2. You may get off track with your eating from time to time. When this happens it can be difficult to get yourself back on track. This can also lead to gaining unwanted pounds. By tracking your calories, you are creating a reference tool. This can help you to get your eating back where you want it to be.

Just go back to your tracking tool and look at what and how you were eating when you were making healthier food and drink choices. Begin to follow that plan to get back to your healthier eating lifestyle.

The Art of Cheating

When deciding whether or not to start on the journey of having a healthier eating lifestyle, one of the concerns can be giving up your favorite foods and how you will survive without them. One of the ways to address this is to incorporate a "cheat day" into your healthier eating plan. This is a day in the week when you can engage in eating some of your favorite foods that you do not have on a daily basis. This usually includes foods like sweet treats, crunchy and salty snacks; as well as, specialty beverages. However, if you are not mindful, a "cheat day" can cause a setback. Here are some tips to have a "cheat day" and stay on track:

1) Plan in advance. Just as you plan out your healthy eating, plan out your cheat day. This day should not be looked at as a day with no limits. The purpose is to be able to enjoy some of your favorite foods, which you no longer have on a regular basis, without going overboard.

2) Stick to the same principles as in a healthier eating lifestyle:

 - Portion control. Be conscious of how much you are eating and drinking.

- Calorie intake. The calories you take in with these foods and drinks may be higher than what you would regularly have. If necessary, track your food and drink so you don't overdo it.

- Water. Even though it's a "cheat day" don't abandon your water intake. It keeps you hydrated and your system flushed.

3) When your "cheat day" is done, make sure to get back on track with your eating plan. Do not delay! When you delay, getting back on track will be more difficult.

Sweet Dreams

Are you getting enough sleep? Not getting enough sleep can be a detriment to your healthier eating lifestyle. Some of the reasons why you may not get enough sleep are working late, watching television (staying up late), screen time (computer), eating late and stress. A lack of sleep causes you to be tired. This, in turn, causes a lack of awareness; which, tends to lead to making unwise choices (especially when it comes to your food and drink). Some of the choices that tend to be made are as follows:

1) Drinking too much coffee and/or soda. When trying to stay alert, there can be a tendency to gravitate to drinking more coffee and/or soda. However, they do not have the nutrients that your body needs. Instead they have caffeine, which is a temporary stimulant. Eventually, with a lack of nutrients and too much caffeine, you will revert back to being tired.

2) Tiredness can also cause you to gravitate towards the foods that you think will help you feel good (your comfort foods). Unfortunately, these foods are usually not healthy foods. Therefore, you may feel energized for a little while, only to feel tired again later.

3) You may also find yourself reaching for those sweet snacks. The sugar will take you up for a moment, but the crash afterward leaves you back where you started, tired.

Getting enough rest is a key element to having a healthier eating lifestyle.

The Joys of Life

The Holidays: It's That Time

The holidays are a wonderful time of the year! They are full of your favorite foods, drinks and desserts. However, you may regret the effects of the holiday meals when they are over. In fact, it is at the end of the holiday season when a number of us begin to check out the nearest fitness facility and try to change and/or get our eating habits back in check. In order to avoid this cycle, the key is to moderate what you do throughout the season, but still be able to enjoy yourself. Believe it or not, this is possible. A few ways to achieve this are:

1) Have light meals and snacks in order to accommodate the extra calories you will be consuming at your holiday events.

2) Prior to heading out to an event, have a protein snack about an hour before arriving. This will help you to feel full, so as not to eat and drink too much.

3) Put gravies, sauces and salad dressings on the side of the plate. Do not pour them on your food! Dip your fork into the gravy/sauce/dressing, and then put the fork into the food. This will minimize the calorie intake and you will have the flavor in every bite.

4) Last, but not least, the dessert table! This is where you can get in the most trouble. The reason for this is everything looks so good and you may want to try a few items instead of sticking to one. When this is the case, take a sample size of the ones that appeal to you instead of a serving size. This enables you to enjoy all of them without overdoing it.

The Holidays: Bottoms Up!

The holidays are full of much merriment! This can have a tendency to include an increased consumption of alcoholic beverages. The calories and sugars in these drinks tend to be high, which can compromise your healthier eating lifestyle. Besides higher calories, there is another effect that these beverages have that can throw you off track. They can slow down your metabolism. That's right! Alcohol has a similar effect on your body that it has on you mentally and physically. Just as it helps you to relax, it also causes your metabolism to relax (slow down). This, in turn, slows down your digestive system.

Another challenge is, as you drink these beverages, you tend to eat more. The slowing down of the metabolism and additional food can be a recipe for disaster. However, you definitely want to be able to enjoy yourself during this season. Therefore, here are a few tips to help you maintain a healthy balance:

49

1) Slow down! Sip your drink. It will last longer and you will drink less.

2) Before you have your next drink, have a glass of water. This will help to keep you hydrated, as well as, help you to consume less alcohol and calories.

3) Minimize the intake of mixed drinks; such as, daiquiris, hurricanes, long island iced teas and cosmopolitans. They taste great, but the sugar levels tend to be high. You may want to try the "skinny" version, if it is available. It will help to reduce the sugar and the calories in your drink.

The goal is to have a great time, without compromising your healthier eating lifestyle and your metabolism!

The Invitation

Throughout the year you may receive invitations to various parties and events. In some cases, you may be asked to bring a dish or a beverage to contribute to the festivities. Sometimes, you may be asked to bring a specific item; and then, there are other times when the choice is yours. Either way, if you're not careful, this invitation can sabotage your healthier eating habits. Upon arrival, you will be faced with all types of food and drink that have been contributed to this gathering. One of the ways to help yourself in these situations is to make your contribution a healthy one. By doing this, you help yourself in various ways:

1) There will be at least one healthy dish you can put on your plate (yours).

2) Your healthy contribution can be a reminder to stay on track as you go around the table making your food and drink choices.

3) By being mindful of your choices, your body may be spared the uncomfortable task of having to recover from overeating.

4) The host/hostess may ask that everyone take their dish home if there is any left over. When this happens, you are able to take home a healthy dish that you can continue to enjoy.

The Sweetest Day

Just as you made it through the holidays, now you are faced with a special day that is focused around food, drinks and sweets. Valentine's Day could be considered the sweetest day of the year in more ways than one. It is a day when we show others how much we love them. It is also a day that can cause a setback if we are not careful. It may involve a special dinner, desserts, alcoholic beverages and specialty beverages; as well as, sweets. The thought can be "it is just for one day". However, depending on how it is handled the effects can last longer than one day. Here are some ways to enjoy this day without having regrets the next day.

1) When you receive chocolate, eat it in moderation. Also, consider sharing it with others.

2) When going out to dinner, plan ahead. If you are able to look at the menu online, decide what you will have before arriving to the restaurant. Plan the rest of your calories

for that day around what you have planned to have for that special dinner. You may want to forfeit some calories during the day to enjoy your food that evening.

3) When it comes to dessert, consider sharing a dessert with someone else. If you have been indulging in sweets throughout the day, think about whether or not dessert should be a part of the plan.

Enjoy the day, but be mindful of how you do it.

Vacation Time

Vacation is a time when your mind and body get a rest from their everyday routine. Sometimes, this rest and relaxation involves trips and cruises, which can mean the availability of an abundance of food and drink. The goal is to have a wonderful time, but to also stay on track with your healthier eating lifestyle. Here are two key principles involved in making this happen:

1) Prepare

Take healthy non-perishable snacks along with you. This will help to deter you from purchasing unhealthy ones. Make some of your snacks protein based like nuts and protein bars. Protein will provide your body with nutrients and a feeling of being full.

2) Plan

When possible, plan your meals in advance. This will help you to monitor your calorie intake. By doing this you are able to maintain your healthier eating by not overindulging.

The goal is to come back from vacation with your body feeling rested and relaxed, not stuffed and bloated.

Staying on Track

Fall/Winter Check In

The seasons are changing and the colder months are moving in. This is a good time to do an assessment on how you are doing with your healthier eating lifestyle. Just as the seasons change, your life may go through changes at this time of year also. The following questions will help you to stay on track with eating healthier through the colder months.

1) How well are you doing at staying on track with your current eating lifestyle?

2) Have there been changes in your schedule that are affecting your eating? If so, now is the time to think about how to make adjustments to maintain your healthier eating habits. (Refer to "Daily Life" and "Busy Life")

3) Are you finding it difficult to maintain a healthier eating lifestyle? If so, then why? You need to know the "why" in order to move forward with figuring out how to create

a plan that works for you. For example, having time to prepare meals may be a challenge. You may want to make your meals in advance, look for "ready to eat" meals in the grocery store or invest in a home delivery service. (Refer to "Busy Life" and "Stabilizing Life")

4) Do you need help staying on track? It may be time to consider tracking your food and/or having an accountability partner. Both of these are great options whether you are beginning your healthier eating lifestyle or have been on it for a period of time. (Refer to "Stabilizing Life")

Fall/Winter Tips

1) This would be a good time to re-visit the chapter entitled "Seasonal Cravings".

2) Watch out for some of the hot beverages that warm you up during the colder months. They tend to be high in calories and sugars. Refer back to the guidelines on pg. 9 (The Specialty Drink Craze).

"After the Holidays"

Yikes! Did you know that quite a few people experience their greatest weight gain during the holidays? Once the festivities are done and life is returning back to normal, it is time to assess how you are doing. If your eating habits have been derailed during the holidays, don't procrastinate about getting back on track. Here are some tips to help you re-establish your healthier eating lifestyle.

1) If you have not tracked your food in the past, this would be a good time to consider doing it. You will want to do this until you get yourself back on track. If you have tracked your food, this is the time when your journal can become a resource for you. In your journal, locate a period of time when you have been on track. Then, begin to mirror those meals, snacks and beverages to get yourself back on course with your healthier eating lifestyle. With your journal, you already have a plan and the best part is it was designed by you.

2) Focus on having protein-based snacks. They provide a feeling of being full and this will help to minimize your calorie intake.

3) Hydrate! If during the holidays you were consuming less water and more drinks that had higher calories, it is time to increase the water and minimize/eliminate the higher calorie drinks.

4) Reduce the sugar! More than likely you increased your sugar intake during the holidays. It is time to get those excess sugars under control.

NOTE: Remember, the spring and summer months will be here before you know it!

Spring/Summer Check In

Spring is in the air! The warmer months of the year are right around the corner. It is time to assess and adjust, if necessary. Just as you switch your closets in the spring of the year, you may need to adjust your eating lifestyle. Here are a few things to consider as you look forward to the warm weather months.

1) How well are you staying on track with your healthier eating lifestyle?

2) Have there been changes in your schedule that are affecting your eating? If so, now is the time to think about how to make adjustments to maintain your healthier eating habits. (Refer to "Daily Life" and "Busy Life")

3) Are you finding it difficult to maintain a healthier eating lifestyle? If so, then why? You need to know the "why" in order to move forward with figuring out how to create a plan that works for you. For example,

during lunch you are on the road most of the time. By the time you get something to eat, it tends to be fast food. In this case, you may want pack a sandwich with a side item; such as vegetables or a piece of fruit. (Refer to "Busy Life" and/or "Stabilizing Life")

4) Do you need help staying on track? It may be time to consider tracking your food and/or having an accountability partner. Both of these are great options whether you are beginning your healthier eating lifestyle or have been on it for a period of time. (Refer to "Stabilizing Life")

Spring/Summer Tips

1) How is your water intake? As the weather begins to get warmer, you may find yourself becoming more dehydrated. Maintaining your hydration level is a key component to maintaining a healthier eating lifestyle.

2) Some of your favorite fruits are in season during the warmer months such as peaches, plums, watermelons, berries and the list goes on. These fruits are like nature's candy. Even though they are natural, they can be high in sugar. Be mindful of this while you are enjoying them.

3) This is a good time to re-visit the chapter entitled, "Lighten Up".